Medication Overload

A Pharmacist's Guide to Managing Medications

Recommendations for Patients and Caregivers

Dr Stephanie Matinpour, PharmD, BCGP

Board Certified Geriatric Pharmacist

©2020 by PillBoxTalk Foundation.
Stephanie Matinpour, Chief Medication Expert

ISBN: 9798617100350

ALL RIGHTS RESERVED
No part of this publication may be reproduced, stored in a retrieval system, or transmitted in any form or by any means, electronic or mechanical, including photocopying, recording, or otherwise, without written permission from PillBoxTalk Foundation.

Created, designed, and produced by PillBoxTalk Foundation.

The information contained herein is provided for educational purposes only and not intended to substitute for a consultation with your primary health-care provider or pharmacist as it pertains to your specific health and medication needs. All patient cases and examples are fictional and all personal health information has been generalized for the purposes of education.

Testimonials

Two of the most important functions that an aging life care professional serves are identifying risk factors for their physically and cognitively impaired clients, and connecting them to the services and supports they need in order to remain healthy and safe in their home. Dr. Matinpour and PillBoxTalk have been an invaluable resource to me on several occasions, when I've identified a client experiencing problems with medication safety or compliance. Her review process is well-informed and thorough, and her follow up with clients, families, and health care providers is always timely and professional. Partnering with a Board Certified Geriatric Pharmacist in the care of my older adult clients has been of tremendous benefit to me, my staff, and of course to those that we serve.

Amy Abrams, MSW/MPH
Education & Outreach Manager
Alzheimer's Association San Diego/Imperial Chapter

Acknowledgements

This book is a compilation of experiences and expertise, and is dedicated to all of the family, friends, colleagues, and patients that have been a part of this medication safety journey!

"A successful partnership between the healthcare provider and patient is one in which each is aware of their role in preventing and managing medication-related problems."

Dr. Stephanie Matinpour, PharmD, BCGP

Table of Contents

Introduction

Medication-Related Problems   **9**

- Medication Related Problems in the Senior Population
- Types of Medication Related Problems
- Assess Your Risk for Medication Related Problems
- Medication Related Problems Assessment Tool

Practical Steps to Reduce Medication-Related Problems   **28**

- Comprehensive Medication Review
- Medication Journals and Tracking
- Visual Aids and Tools for Proper Administration of Medications
- Questions to ask your Provider or Pharmacist

Proper Storage and Disposal of Medications   **35**

- Medication Storage Tips
- Proper Disposal of Medications
- Disposing of Needles and Sharps Containers

Saving Money on Your Medications   **43**

- Splitting Tablets for the Wrong Reasons
- Skipping doses
- Medications from Family and Friends
- Purchasing from Foreign Companies
- Purchasing over the Internet
- Generics: They're Usually Cheaper!
- Combination Products
- Don't Take Unnecessary Medication
- Split Tablets Correctly
- Manufacturer Coupons
- Drug Companies' Patient Assistance Programs

Over-the-Counter Remedies and Herbal Supplements   **53**

- Over-the-Counter Approval Process
- Natural Supplements
- Understanding Interactions with Prescription Medications

Conversations with Your Healthcare Provider(s)   **57**

- Conversations with Your Physician
- Conversations with Your Pharmacist
- Conversations with Your Support System

Ask the Pharmacist: Expertise from a Clinical Pharmacist   **65**

introduction

As the Baby Boomers begin to enter their golden years, many have dreams and aspirations of living an active and healthy life well into retirement age. Most of us envision a life of low stress and lots of free time to spend with our families. What we don't plan on is the reality of chronic disease states and of multiple medications running our lives.

While many Americans are living much longer lives, we are living them with multiple chronic conditions such as diabetes, high blood pressure, and high cholesterol. Each of these disease states on its own is very complex, and when you add into the mix multiple medications, doctors, and pharmacies filling prescriptions, you have a higher risk of medication-related problems.

Clinical Pharmacists are licensed pharmacists highly trained in the proper use and monitoring of medications, specifically those in the senior population. From Alzheimer's disease to osteoporosis, we work with our patients to ensure that they are getting the most benefit from the medications they are taking, while continually evaluating their medication regimen to ensure that the medications our patients take are safe and effective.

We work with patients and caregivers in order to maintain independence in the home setting, while navigating the complex healthcare model we are currently working within. On average, patients see three physicians per year and utilize multiple pharmacies to fill their prescriptions. Clinical Pharmacists serve as personal pharmacists to patients and their caregivers, guiding them through the medications they are prescribed to attempt to avoid any medication-related problems.

As a vital member of the healthcare team, the Clinical Pharmacist is an additional resource to guide patients and their caregivers to help them achieve their best health. As medication experts, Clinical Pharmacists are Licensed Pharmacists working with the patient's physician and providers to recommend appropriate drug therapy.

This book is a guide to those looking for assistance in understanding their medications as well as the questions that they should be asking their physicians and healthcare providers. My hope is that it provides you with the tools and perspectives you need to be your own medication safety advocate.

Dr Stephanie Matinpour, PharmD, BCGP

Founder, Executive Director PillBoxTalk

www.pillboxtalk.com

LET'S GET STARTED!

MEDICATION-RELATED PROBLEMS: WHAT IS YOUR RISK?

A **medication-related problem (MRP)** is an event or situation involving medications that cause you harm or prolong, perhaps worsen a current condition. A medication-related problem can range from harmless to deadly. Basically, a medication-related problem is anything "bad" that happens to your body as a result of taking a medication or several medications. A medication-related problem can be as simple as stomach upset or severe enough to cause death. Most medication-related problems are not detected, because people do not look at medications as a potential cause of their problems.

Medication-related problems prevent patients from getting positive results from the medications that they are taking. They waste valuable time and money, because patients end up taking medications that don't work for them, or they need additional medications to offset the harm caused by the original medications. This often leads to extra visits to the doctors office or emergency room.

Drug therapy in seniors presents multiple clinical challenges due to age and disease-related alterations in drug absorption, distribution, metabolism, and elimination. Adverse drug effects are frequently the source of problems associated with aging such as confusion, impaired motor function, and depression. Good medication management in the senior population involves identifying and resolving adverse drug events rather than treating them with additional drugs.

One of my patients once asked me, **"Why in the world are we taking so many medications these days? Our parents and their parents never took half the pills we take, and they seemed to make out okay."** Well, there is not a very simple question to answer, as there are many things different about our world today compared to 20 or 30 years ago. There are many theories about this, including that the American diet has greatly affected our health outcomes. However, the more obvious observation is that people are living much longer today than they did 30 years ago. Living longer with chronic conditions often leads to multiple medications.

Studies have found that those with chronic conditions often do not take their medications properly, which can lead to negative consequences to both the patient and the health care system. Due to this and other factors, medication-related problems are the leading cause of accidental death in the United States, even above motor vehicle accidents.

A study released by the American Pharmaceutical Association estimates that drug misuse costs the U.S. economy more than $177 billion every year in hospital and long-term care admissions. Physician and emergency department visits added to these treatment costs, and resulted in 218,000 deaths in 2000. The study linked these healthcare and societal costs to adverse drug reactions, drug interactions, inappropriate dosage, and failure to receive medications. Most of these costs and hospitalizations can be prevented by understanding more about medication related problems and how they affect your health.

Medication Related Problems in the Senior Population

In the general population, medication-related problems may prolong or worsen an existing condition and may also cause other additional health problems. In addition, the senior population is at an increased risk of developing medication related problems for several reasons.

First, the process of aging causes changes to the body and affects how we respond to medications. For example, as we age we often see a decrease in water intake and increase in body fat composition. These two factors alone can greatly affect how medications are absorbed into the bloodstream and metabolized in the body. In addition, as we age, our kidney and liver functions often decrease, which can affect how medications are eliminated from our body.

In addition, older adults are also more likely to be taking multiple medications, leading to an increased risk of medication interactions. They are also more likely to have chronic medical conditions that can cause the body to respond differently to medications than the average person. In addition, as we age, we are more likely to have poor eyesight, which could affect the ability to read and understand prescription labels, as well as poor grip strength, which could affect the ability to open medication bottles. Furthermore, age-related memory challenges, or even dementia, make it difficult for patients to remember to take their medications properly.

When medications are first studied for Federal Drug Administration (FDA) approval, the agency often does not monitor how the medications will affect the senior population or those with chronic conditions. Therefore, problems specific to those with multiple medications or chronic conditions are usually not identified until **after** the medications have been approved for the general population.

Types of Medication Related Problems

Medication-related problems can generally be put into three buckets:

1. Not using enough of the medication (Underuse)
- Results in a medical condition that is not being treated
- Dose of the medication is too low
- Unsure of how to take the medication properly
- Not taking the medication for a Financial or Functional reason
- Emotional/psychological barriers (fear, embarrassment, memory issues)
- Using an incorrect medication
- Using a medication that is not the best medication to treat the problem

2. Using too much of the medication (Overuse)
- No reason for the medication
- Dose is too high
- Duplicate medications
- Take too much of the medication
  - Due to error
  - Due to technique
- Wrong drug for the condition being treated
- Not the best medication to treat the problem

3. **Side effects of medications**
    - Incorrect medication
    - Allergy
    - Drug interaction
    - Food
    - Disease
    - Other medication (prescription, non-prescription, and/or herbal)
    - Side effect of normal dose or high dose
    - Rare adverse reaction

Let's look at examples of **UNDERUSE OF MEDICATIONS**

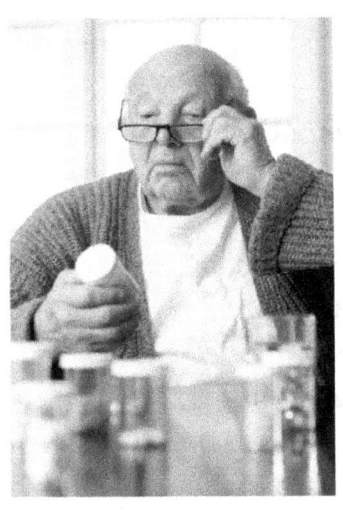*Larry has high cholesterol and his doctor has prescribed a starting (low-dose) statin medication to take every evening, starting immediately. Larry forgets to go to the lab in 6 weeks as instructed by his physician. Because he "feels fine", he keeps taking the low-dose statin and figures he'll just follow-up with his doctor in 6 months.*

In this example, we see the use of a common medication for high cholesterol. Studies have shown this medication to be extremely effective in lowering cholesterol quickly and preventing heart attacks. However, we also know that this class of medication has some common side effects that can be tolerated over time, *if* we slowly titrate (that is, if we reduce) the dose to an amount appropriate for that specific patient. That's what Larry's doctor was attempting to do by appropriately checking his blood work in 6 weeks in order to make sure the medication was working properly.

When Larry skips the lab work and continues to take the low "starting dose", he isn't properly protected from a potential heart attack, and is also wasting money on a medication that may not be effective for him. It's important to make sure that, once you get a new prescription from your doctor, you follow-up with ordered lab work and appointments to ensure you are on the appropriate dose of medication.

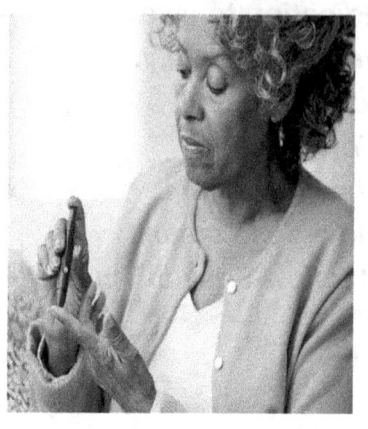
Marge was just diagnosed with Type 2 Diabetes, and her doctor started her on Metformin (Glucophage®), 250mg twice a day. She's been very compliant about taking her medication, and checking her blood sugars four times a day. However she is not seeing a decrease in the blood sugar value.

In this example, we see a newly diagnosed patient with diabetes Type 2 being, who was prescribed a common medication for this chronic condition. What is not common in this scenario is the starting dose. This would be considered an extremely low starting dose, which would only be considered if Marge had serious kidney dysfunction and there were no other medication options for her. Often with newly diagnosed diabetic patients, after implementing lifestyle modifications, starting Metformin is the next step; however, it's important that the patient is started on the right dose to get the blood sugars under control as quickly and safely as possible.

It's important to contact your provider to ensure your dose is appropriate if you haven't seen your blood sugars in the normal range within the first one to two weeks. It's also important to keep a daily log of your sugars that you can share with your physician or pharmacist. Most glucose monitors available on the market right now allow for results to be automatically saved; you

can then send those results electronically. If you don't know how to utilize this functionality on your monitor, ask your provider at your next visit, or simply utilize the blood glucose tracker within our **MedTracker** journal available on our website.
www.pillboxtalk.com

Let's look at examples of **OVERUSE OF MEDICATIONS**

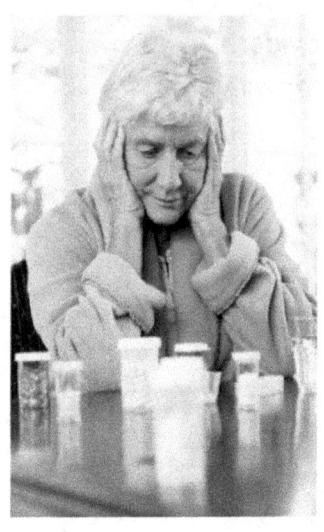
Patty has arthritis and has been taking Advil for her pain. The pain is getting worse, so she sees her doctor, who recommends that she try Aleve, which Patty can buy over the counter. Patty forgets to tell her doctor that she's already taking Advil, and, being in severe pain, she takes both medications for a few weeks. She then develops stomach pains and ends up in the emergency room with a bleeding ulcer.

In this example, we see an overuse of two medications from the same class. Aleve (naproxen) and Advil (ibuprofen) are both in a class of medications called non-steroidal-anti-inflammatory-drugs, also known as "NSAIDs". This class of medications is a commonly used over-the-counter treatment for pain and reduces inflammation. Taking just one of these types of medications can increase your risk of a stomach ulcer, if you take too much of the medication or for too long.

Therefore, when Patty unknowingly takes two of the same types of medications, she puts herself at a very high risk of being hospitalized with a bleeding stomach ulcer. This is why it is so important to review all your medications, including those purchased over the counter, with your doctor or pharmacist. In this example of **Over Use of Medications**, it is again important to check with your pharmacist or physician!

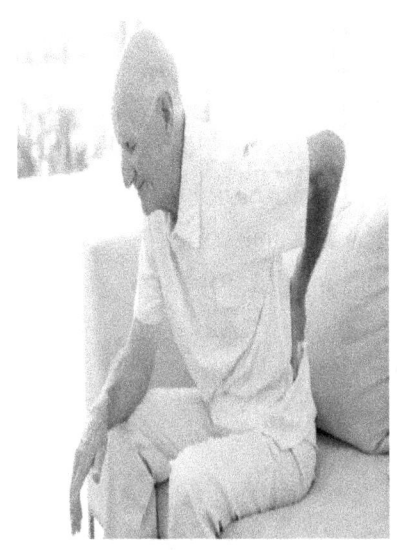
Joe has back pain, so his doctor prescribed pain medication to take every 6 hours, around the clock, for the next 7 to 10 days. After starting the prescribed medication, the pain returns after 4 hours, and so Joe starts taking Tylenol every 4 hours, along with the prescription pain medication. Several weeks later, Joe notices the whites of his eyes have a yellow color.

In this scenario, we see a person with chronic back pain, who has tried taking over-the-counter pain relievers with no luck. He does the appropriate thing and schedules an appointment with his physician. In this particular case, the physician prescribes a common pain medication called Norco (hydrocodone-acetaminophen). Unfortunately, what gets missed in the communication of this new additional medication is that each tablet contains acetaminophen, which is also the active ingredient in Tylenol.

While most understand that Tylenol (acetaminophen) is considered a very "safe" over-the-counter pain reliever, what is not commonly communicated is that your body can only process a certain amount of acetaminophen in 24 hours. When we exceed that amount and take too much acetaminophen, it affects our liver and can lead to liver toxicity, which is what we are seeing in this scenario. This is why it is so important to let your Provider or Pharmacist know of any over the counter or herbal supplements that you are taking. In recent years we have seen a significant issue with patients having liver toxicity secondary to acetaminophen exposure, regardless of age.

The recommended daily maximum amount of acetaminophen in a healthy individual is ~4,000mg per 24 hours. However, if you already have liver issues or drink alcohol that number could be significantly less. Liver toxicity from acetaminophen overdosage can be reversed if caught early enough, but can be fatal if not identified early on. Again, when in doubt ask your pharmacist!

Let's look at examples of **MEDICATIONS SIDE EFFECTS**

Janet has had two falls in the past two weeks, and she often wakes up in the middle of the night and forgets where she is. She has high blood pressure, and her doctor recently increased her medication. She also bought some Tylenol PM to help her sleep at night.

In this scenario, we have a person with a history of falls and some memory issues. She also recently had her blood pressure medication increased by her physician, and purchased an over-the-counter remedy to help her sleep at night.

First, let's discuss the increased blood pressure medication. As we age, we are often susceptible to a condition called orthostatic hypotension, which means that, when we stand from a sitting position, the blood flow to our brain isn't as quick as it used to be, and so we can get light-headed, dizzy and possibly risk falling. This is possibly what's happening for Janet.

Another possibility is that Janet may have what we refer to as "white-coat hypertension". White-coat hypertension is something we commonly see when a patient is anxious or nervous at the doctor's office, and so their blood pressure is abnormally elevated just for that visit. They may have "normal" or stable blood pressure in the home setting; therefore, increasing the medication dose at the doctor's appointment can lead to the side effect of hypotension, or blood pressure that is too low, which can lead to dizziness or falls. This is why we encourage our patients to check and to document their blood pressure daily at home first thing in the morning.

Most home-use blood pressure monitors have the capability of storing past blood pressure readings so that you can share with your physician. If you don't know how to utilize this functionality, ask your provider at your next visit or simply utilize the blood pressure tracker within our **MedTracker** journal available on our website. www.pillboxtalk.com

The other issue Janet is having is related to her memory; specifically, she is using medications that could be contributing to medication-induced dementia. The medication that she recently purchased over the counter was Tylenol PM. Again, this is a medication that you can easily purchase over the counter without a prescription or recommendation from the pharmacist.

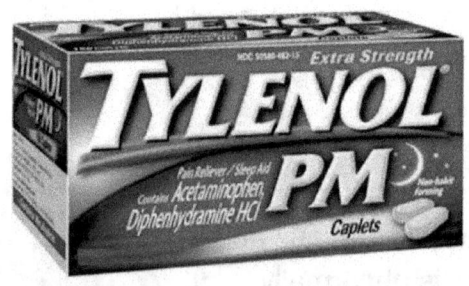

Tylenol PM is a combination medication that contains both acetaminophen (for pain) and diphenhydramine (to help with sleep). The amount of acetaminophen in each caplet of Tylenol PM is not really enough to treat any aches or pains that might be keeping someone up at night. So if aches and pains are the reason you're having trouble sleeping, it's better to just take acetaminophen alone, and not as a combination medication, so that you can be sure you are getting the appropriate dose.

Diphenhydramine is also the active ingredient in Benadryl, and the main side effect of this medication is drowsiness. This is the reason Tylenol PM helps you fall asleep: it's simply the side effect of the medication. The problem we run into with this type of medication is that, as we age, the way diphenhydramine works in our body changes. It can linger longer, and can cause us to be sleepy or groggy even after we have woken up the next morning. This could be significantly contributing to Janet's falls in the past couple of weeks.

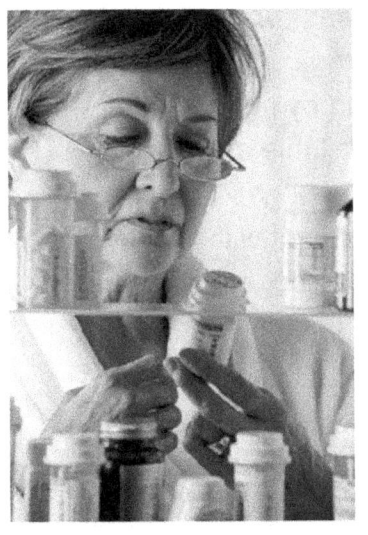

Irma has been taking medication for depression for a few months with no improvement. She doesn't drive and doesn't want to bother the family to take her to the doctor again. She purchases St. John's Wort at the local grocery store after her cousin recommended it. After taking it for a few days she feels groggy, nauseous, and weak.

In this scenario, Irma has a diagnosis of depression, and was appropriately placed on an antidepressant medication by her physician. Like many seniors, she relies on her family and friends to get her to her medical appointments and trusts their opinions and recommendations when it comes to her health.

When someone is first diagnosed with depression and placed on a medication, it can take sometimes up to 3 months for the physician to determine the appropriate dose of the medication, based on depression screenings and side effect management. It's important to follow your physician's instructions when starting these medications, and to not stop abruptly without discussing it with your provider, as this can lead to adverse side effects.

Another issue we see is the drug-drug interaction with some "natural" supplements and commonly prescribed antidepressants. In this particular scenario, Irma is already on an antidepressant prescribed by her physician. Instead of contacting the provider when she feels it "isn't working", she takes an over the counter supplement recommended by her family. St. John's Wort is a common supplement available at most health food stores, and while it does have some beneficial uses, it's also possible for medications like this to interact with others and to cause significant health issues with very negative outcomes.

Assess Your Risk For Medication-Related Problems

In summary, **medication-related problems** prevent you from getting positive results from the medications that you are taking, and often waste time and money, because:

- The medications don't work.
- You need different/more medications or treatments, because the original medications have caused harm.
- Medication related problems cause extra visits to the doctor or the emergency room.
- Medication related problems may prolong or worsen the original condition.
- Medication related problems may cause other, new health problems.

The question then becomes, "At what point are you at risk for medication-related problems?" For example, when should you start to ask questions of your healthcare provider to verify if certain medications are really necessary; and, better yet, are you taking your medications in the most optimal way to achieve the goal of therapy?

Medication-related problems can cause, aggravate, or contribute to common and costly geriatric problems. Clinical Pharmacists identify and prevent medication related problems through careful evaluation and monitoring of patients' drug regimens.

One of the most important things to ask yourself is, "What increases my risk for a medication-related problem?" There are a variety of assessments out there, including the one we will describe now. In general, ask yourself **Do I...**

- Take **5** or more **medications**?"
- Take **12** or more medication **doses** per day?"
- Change my medication regimen four or more times during the past **year**?"
- Have **3** or more medical **conditions**?"
- **Forget** to take **medications**?"
- Take drugs that require **intense drug monitoring** (such as a blood thinner)?"

Before taking the following assessment, sit down and review **all** of the medications you take, which includes those prescribed by your doctor and over-the-counter supplements. Think about those medications you only take for headaches or backaches and how often you really take them. Also consider any dietary supplements, such as fish oil or green tea, which can have significant interactions with some medications.

If you are 65 years or older and answer **"YES"** to more than three of the questions below, you may be at risk for medication related problems.

Risk Factor	Circle One	
Do you currently take 5 or more medications?	Yes	No
Do you take 12 or more medication doses each day?	Yes	No
Are you currently taking medications for 3 or more medical problems?	Yes	No
Have your medications or the instructions on how to take them been changed 4 or more times this past year?	Yes	No
Does more than 1 physician prescribe medications for you on a regular basis?	Yes	No
Do you get your prescriptions filled at more than 1 pharmacy?	Yes	No
Does someone else bring any of your medications to your home for you (such as a delivery person from the pharmacy, a spouse, a partner, a friend, or a neighbor)?	Yes	No
Is it difficult for you to follow your medication regimen, and/or do you sometimes choose not to?	Yes	No
Of all your medications, are there any that you do not know the reason for taking?	Yes	No

There are many ways to help ensure that you are taking your medication properly. Let's Get Started

PRACTICAL STEPS TO REDUCE MEDICATION-RELATED PROBLEMS

Using your medications the right way is very important to your health. The proper use of medications not only helps you to get the full benefit from those you take, but also reduces your chances of having side effects and problems that could occur from taking medications the wrong way.

Studies show that patients who have a good relationship with their health care providers are better at communicating issues that they are having. It's important to be clear with your healthcare provider about issues and barriers that prevent you from taking your medications properly. When you are having trouble taking your medications properly, it's important to communicate that to your healthcare provider so a plan can be developed that works for your situation.

Comprehensive Medication Review

A comprehensive medication review by a Clinical Pharmacist is the first step in assuring your medications have been assessed regardless of provider or specialist. One of the main objectives of having a comprehensive medication review by a Clinical Pharmacist is to provide you with a personal medication action plan that you can utilize to track your progress and to follow up on a scheduled basis.

This step ensures that you don't miss any appointments or lab work that may be necessary for medications that need regular monitoring. Setting up a consultation with a Clinical Pharmacist is a great first step to ensuring that your medication action plan is reviewed annually and kept up-to-date.

The medication action plan is a tool used by Clinical Pharmacists to assist you and your physician in managing your chronic conditions. The medication action plan can be thought of as a road map to guide you at your physician appointments and when tracking your goals.

Medication Journals and Tracking

One of the easiest things you can start with is a medication journal or record that you carry with you at all times. A medication journal is simply a list of all of your current medications. The medication journal should include, at minimum, the name of and instructions for each medication. It's also helpful to have the prescribing physician's name and contact information, and to include any allergies that you might have to medications. You may also want to include any medications you have tried in the past, but no longer take, either because they didn't work for you or because you had an intolerance to them. This is extremely helpful in preventing any duplications in therapy or adverse events. You can track your medications and compliance utilizing our **MedTracker** journal available on our website. www.pillboxtalk.com

Visual Aids for Proper Administration of Medications

After you have sorted out your medications and organized your medication list, it's important to remember to actually take your medications! Many devices and systems are available in the market today to assist you in organizing and taking your medications. Here is a summary of a few of the options currently available on the market to assist with medication administration.

Medication Boxes

A number of medication boxes are available on the market. The most commonly used reminder devices are pill boxes that organize pills by the days and times to be taken. These pill boxes simplify multiple medications that have to be taken daily and help you to remember to take your medications each day. Using pillboxes along with a calendar or medication journal can serve as a double-check system to help you remember to take your medications daily.

More complex pill boxes are electronic and have alarms or beepers that can be programmed for the specific time a medication needs to be taken. These types of pill boxes can be useful for someone who has memory problems, but who is still able to hear the beeping of an alarm.

Medication Reminder Services

With advances in technology, more and more medication reminder systems are utilizing email and text messaging. Several different websites are currently available to set up yourself, for free, to either call or text you when it's time to take your medications. However, please be aware that you may be charged for text messages. Alternatively, you can just set the alarm on your smartphone.

Visual and Sensory Aids

Along with pill boxes to organize your medications, visual aids are just as important to remind you of proper administration once at home. Many people consider themselves "visual learners", and so a picture, to them, is worth a thousand words. Ask your pharmacist for any brochures, flyers, print-outs or charts that they may have to help you understand how to properly take your medication.

Most pharmacies have the capability to print your prescription labels and instructions in **LARGE FONT**. So if it's hard for you to read the small print on the label, please ask your pharmacist to provide you with literature in a larger font.

Many of our patients have low or no vision as they advance in age, making sensory aids essential in assuring proper administration of medications. Most pill boxes manufactured in the United States have braille symbols imprinted on the medication containers. Also, there are now devices such as "talking pill boxes" and insulin meters, which can tell you exactly what medication you are taking and what your blood sugar readings are.

One of the tools created for my clients with visual or memory issues is the SmartMedTag. The tags are used to assist those taking multiple doses of medications throughout the day. The SmartMedTag is simply attached to the medication bottle to track medication adherence.

These are just a few of the tools to help you reduce medication errors in the home setting. The key to reducing your risk is communication and your last safety guard before heading home on a new medication is your pharmacist. Therefore, **always ask your doctor or pharmacist about new medications.**

Questions to Ask your Provider or Pharmacist

It's important that you always ask the following questions every time you get a new or change in your current medication regimen:

What is the name of my medication?
Learn the names of all your medications and why you are taking each one.

What is it supposed to do?
Understand the goal of your medications, and what the outcome should be.

When and how should I take my medication?
- Should I take this medication on an empty stomach or with food?
- How often should I take it?
- At what time of day should I take it?

What if I forget to take my medication?
Try to follow the directions as closely as possible. And if you miss a dose, *do not* take a double dose. Instead, ask your pharmacist for his or her advice about a missed dose when you have the prescription order filled. You should know the answer to this question before you need it!

How long should I take it?
You could bring on a serious health problem if you don't take all your medication, or if you continue to take some medications for too long. Your doctor should indicate the length of time with your

prescription order. Ask your pharmacist about over-the-counter (OTC) medications.

What about taking other medications or drinking alcohol at the same time?
Your prescription and OTC medications may interact with other drugs and cause a harmful effect. Certain foods or alcohol also may interact with drug products. Never begin taking a new medication without asking your pharmacist if it will interact with alcohol, foods, or other medicines.

Now that you've identified them, how do you dispose of unwanted medications? Let's get started!

PROPER STORAGE & DISPOSAL OF MEDICATIONS

Where do you keep your medications? Are they in different places, with some in the medicine cabinet, some in the kitchen, and some in the bedroom or elsewhere? As a parent, grandparent, or family member, it's important that you organize and keep track of the location of your loved one's medications. After all, you will want to know where a particular medication is when you or someone else needs to find it. And you will want to keep your medication secure, so that a child, teenager, or even a stranger cannot access them. In this way, you can help prevent an accidental injury, as well as do your part to stop the possible abuse of prescription medications.

The first step in getting organized is to take a look at all the medications you have. You should try to do this type of inventory every six months, or at least once a year. Start by checking the expiration date on the bottles; you don't want to take any chances with a medicine that no longer works the way it's supposed to. Check the expiration date for eye drops and ear drops, too. They may no longer be effective and, worse, could be a breeding ground for bacteria or fungus.

Also, look for medications that are discolored, dried out, crumbling, or show other signs that they are past their prime. In addition, look for leftover prescription medications from a previous illness or condition. You will want to discard these, since you should never try to treat yourself, or anyone else for that matter, with a prescription medication. Your symptoms might seem similar to those you've had before, but the cause could be different, or the medication may not be the right one this time around.

Now that you've identified the medications you want to keep, the next step is to find a safe place to keep them. You'll want to store your medication in an area that is convenient, but is also cool and dry, since heat and humidity can damage medications.

That's why a bathroom is not a good place to keep your medications, unless you are able to keep the room well ventilated. However, the bathroom medicine cabinet is an ideal place to keep other items, such as bandages, tweezers, gauze, cotton balls, scissors, and other products that aren't affected by heat or humidity.

If there are children around, you might also want to find an area where you can lock up your medications. A cabinet or a drawer with a lock on it would work. It's also an excellent idea to lock up any controlled substances that have been prescribed for you. As theft and abuse of prescription medications is a serious problem. These include medications such as hydromorphone (Dilaudid®), oxycodone (OxyContin® and Percocet®), hydrocodone (Vicodin®), and alprazolam (Xanax®).

You can play a large and very helpful role in keeping these powerful medications out of the hands of those who shouldn't have them. Since it is dangerous as well as illegal for anyone else to use a controlled substance prescribed for you, a locked storage area should be found, in order to help keep a stranger or someone else from gaining access to them.

Medication Storage Tips

Here are some suggestions that can help you to be smarter about storing and using your medications:

- Keep your medications separate from those of your spouse or other family members, for instance, on a different shelf or at least on a separate side of a shelf. This will make it less likely that you take the wrong ones by mistake.

- You may find it helpful to have a countertop or tabletop near where you keep your medication, so that you can open the bottle with it resting on the flat surface. In case you drop your pill, it will land on the tabletop and not be lost down the drain or on the floor. Just be sure not to leave your medication bottles out on the counter afterwards.

- Good lighting near where you store your medications will help you make sure you are taking the right medication. *Never take medications in the dark.*

- Keep the medication in the bottle it came in. The amber color protects the medication from light. You will also have the information right on the bottle, telling what the medication is and how often to take it. The label will also have the phone number of the pharmacy so you can call when it is time for a refill.

- Never mix different medications in the same bottle. You might end up taking the wrong one by mistake.

- Keep the lids on your pill bottles tightly closed. A cap can't be childproof if it's not fastened correctly.

- If there is cotton in the pill bottle when you first open it, remove the cotton and throw it away. The cotton can absorb moisture and affect the medication that is inside.

It's important to store medications at room temperature, and not in the refrigerator or freezer, unless the mediation specifically needs to be stored at a cooler temperature. Refrigerated medications may remain potent for several days if extreme heat is avoided.

For example, most insulin vials can be used for at least 28 days if kept at room temperature. If refrigeration is recommended, keep the medication as cool as possible but avoid freezing. If you have any concerns about leaving a medication at a temperature that is not appropriate, discussion with the pharmacist will be needed to determine if and when the medication needs to be replaced.

Proper Disposal of Medications

Now that we have reviewed the proper storage and review of our medications for expiration dates, what do you do with those out-dated or unneeded medications? How should you dispose of them?

Most drugs can be thrown in the trash, but you should take certain precautions before tossing them out. A growing number of "take-back" programs offer another safe way to dispose of your medications.

- **Follow disposal instructions** on the drug label or patient information that comes with your medications. **Never** flush prescription drugs down the toilet unless instructed by your pharmacist or physician.

- If available in your area, use a drug take-back program that allows you to bring unused drugs to a central location for disposal.

- Call your city or county government trash and recycling service to see if your city has such a program. The federal Drug Enforcement Agency, working with state and local law enforcement, sponsors National Prescription Drug Take Back Days throughout the U.S. For more about this, go to http://www.deadiversion.usdoj.gov

If disposal instructions are not given on the drug label, and there are no take-back programs available in your area, here are some tips to properly dispose of medicines in the trash:

1. Take them out of their original containers and remove or conceal any personal information.
2. Mix the medication with something non-toxic, but that with a definite odor, such as used coffee grounds or kitty litter. The medication will be less appealing to children and pets, and unrecognizable to people who may go through your trash.
3. Put the mixture in a sealable bag, an empty can, or other container. This will prevent the medication from leaking or breaking through a garbage bag.

Some Additional Tips

- Before throwing out a drug container, scratch out personal information on the label like your name, the drug name, etc. This will help protect your privacy and your health information.
- Do not give medications to friends. A drug that works for you could be dangerous for someone else.
- If you are not sure how to dispose of your meds, talk to your pharmacist.
- The same steps above can also be used to dispose of over-the-counter and herbal products.

Disposing of Needles and Sharps Containers

The number of people with insulin dependent diabetes is on the rise; therefore, it's important to understand the proper disposal of syringes and needles.

Many states prohibit the disposal of "sharps waste", including needles, syringes, and lancets, in the regular trash. Sharps waste poses a risk to trash collectors, who may accidentally get stuck by a needle, syringe or lancet and be exposed to a disease. Your children, pets, domestic workers, and janitors may also be at risk of a needle stick if needles are improperly stored or disposed of. Used sharps could:

- injure people,
- spread germs, or
- spread serious disease like HIV/AIDS, hepatitis, and tetanus

Sharps should *not* be:

- thrown in the trash,
- flushed down the toilet, or
- placed in recycling containers.

Put Sharps Waste in its Place!

- Ask your healthcare provider or pharmacist if they take back used needles, lancets, and syringes.
- Take your used needles, lancets, and syringes to drop-off collection sites or household hazardous waste facilities.
- Consider using a "mail-back" service for proper disposal. For a list of mail-back service companies, visit your state's Department of Public Health website's home page for drop off locations (fees might apply for this service).

IDENTIFY EXPIRED OR UNUSED MEDICATIONS 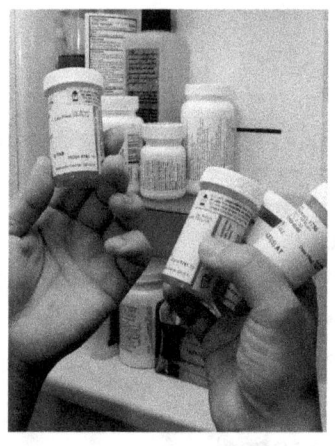	**SCRATCH OUT OR MARK OUT ANY PERSONAL INFORMATION ON THE LABEL** 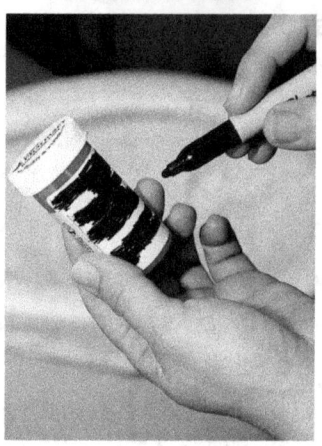
MAKE MEDICATION UNPALATABLE BY MIXING WITH WATER AND SOMETHING NON-TOXIC, SUCH AS KITTY LITTER OR COFFEE GROUNDS 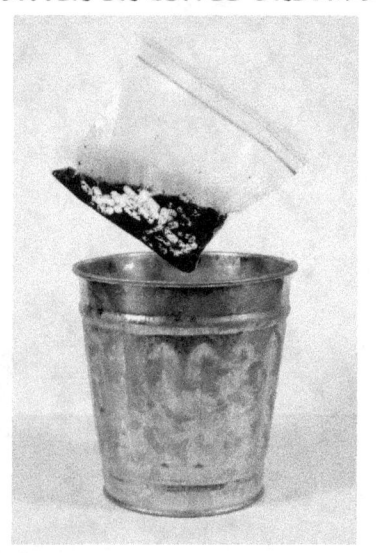	**DISPOSE OF MEDICATIONS CLOSE TO TRASH PICK-UP TIME OR DROP OFF AT A LOCAL COLLECTION SITE** 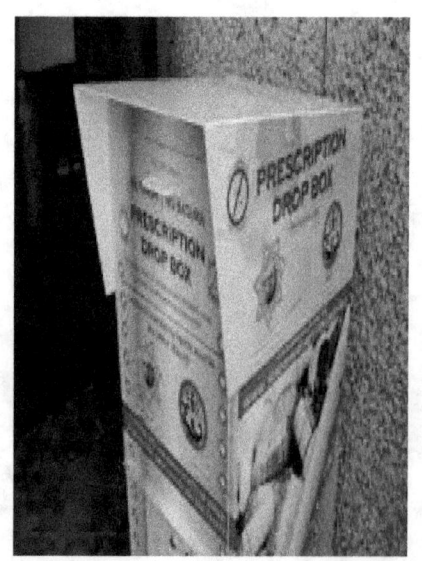

SAVING MONEY ON YOUR MEDICATIONS

Let's face it, staying healthy can cost money! Eating fresh fruits and vegetables is typically more expensive than buying frozen and canned. Purchasing organic foods costs more than buying the same foods full of chemicals and preservatives. And trying to prevent disease, or treat and cure health conditions, can be costly when it comes to using certain medications.

Over the years practicing pharmacists and medical professionals have seen individuals struggle with this financial dilemma. Sometimes patients are having to choose between their much needed medications and the basic necessities of life, like food and shelter. It is amazing the lengths that individuals will go to in order to make their medications more affordable. Some examples are:

- Splitting tablets for the wrong reasons
- Taking daily medications every other day
- Taking medications given to them from family or friends
- Purchasing medications from foreign companies
- Purchasing medications over the Internet

Although each of these scenarios may save individuals much needed money. However, in the long run the cost to one's health and to their pocketbooks, could far exceed the immediate savings. Let's dive a little deeper into each of these potentially dangerous scenarios.

Splitting tablets for the wrong reasons

Medication is prescribed in specific doses in order to achieve a specific outcome. Let's look at an example. Say a patient has high blood pressure and has been prescribed; lisinopril, at a dose of 20 mg per day. If the patient decides on his or her own to only take half the dose, what would be the result? You got it! The blood pressure would rise, and possibly, depending on the level, put the patient at risk for a heart attack or stroke. Not exactly saving money overall, is it?

Every other day (skipping doses)

The end result of this scenario is basically the same as the scenario above: putting the patient at risk for negative health outcomes. If you're not able to afford to take your medication in the way that your doctor prescribed, please discuss your concerns with your provider or pharmacist, so that they can look into other options for you. For example, lifestyle changes, generic medication, or other appropriate medications covered by your insurance policy.

Medications from family and friends

Using these medications is not the best choice for several reasons. First, it can be dangerous. Frequently, we see people getting confused about medications that look the same. There are numerous little, white, round tablets that all look very much alike. Similar sounding names, for example hydroxyzine and hydralazine sound very much alike, and so are often confused.

Second, in the case of controlled substances, giving medication to another person, or taking another person's medication is illegal. Did you know that controlled medications, by law, should only be taken by the person they are prescribed to, and that the labeling even states, "Federal Law Prohibits the Transfer of this drug to any other person than for whom it was prescribed"? Bottom line: taking other people's medications is never a good idea!

Purchasing from foreign companies

This, too, is not a good idea, even though it can save a lot of money in the short term. The reason this is not safe is because of the uncertain quality of the substance. In the United States, the Food and Drug Administration (FDA) regulates how medications are brought to market, sold and stored, and they enact these regulations to protect the public. Not all foreign countries have this oversight with regard to medications.

Because this oversight may be absent elsewhere, as a consumer, if you purchase medications from other countries, you may be receiving medications that have been stored improperly, possibly having lost their potency. The end result could be similar to that of pill splitting or alternating days, reducing the medication's effectiveness and putting individuals at risk for complications. As in our blood pressure example, this could be the risk of heart attack and stroke.

Another possibility when purchasing foreign medications is that they might be adulterated. This means that the medication may be contaminated, sub-potent, or counterfeit. And yes, this really happens!

Back in 2006, 115 people died in Panama after taking a cough syrup that was made with inexpensive diethylene glycol in place of the more expensive, safe ingredient, glycerin. And in the U.S. in 2007 and 2008, there were 149 deaths due to a contaminated ingredient introduced during the manufacturing process of heparin, an intravenous product designed to thin the blood, that was manufactured in China and then exported to a U.S. drug manufacturer. This last incident generated much criticism of the drug manufacturer and the FDA, for not having physically traveled to China in a timely manner to conduct a thorough inspection of the Chinese manufacturing plant.

As you can see, not all countries have processes in place to ensure strict manufacturing practices that are designed to deliver safe products and to protect the intended consumer. Because of this, unless you do extensive research yourself into the manufacturing regulations of other companies and countries that supply medications, you are probably better off not purchasing outside the U.S.

Purchasing over the Internet

Sometimes you can save substantial money by buying your medications online; however, if you choose this supply source, you'll need to do some research to make sure that the supplier is legitimate and follows safe practices. Concerns with purchasing through the Internet include: some suppliers may claim to be pharmacies, but are not, or that they are not licensed to dispense medications within the U.S.

Other concerns are that some companies may not protect your personal information, for example your credit card information, health history, or medications history. Additional concerns are that medications may be counterfeit, too weak or too strong, contaminated, expired, or not stored or shipped appropriately to protect the integrity of the product.

In order to protect your personal information and your health, if you choose this online route of obtaining your medications, you must know the source of the medication (for example, their licensing, the manufacturing location) and how that the seller as well as the manufacturer will protect your personal and health information.

Now that we've eliminated these risky cost-saving approaches, you might be feeling discouraged and wondering how you can possibly afford your medications. There are still things you *can* do that can help you save your hard earned money!

Generics: They're usually cheaper!

First, let's educate you on brand versus generic medications. All medications have been assigned a generic name. When a drug company spends millions of dollars and many years on developing a new drug, once it's approved by the FDA, they are allowed exclusive rights to sell the drug under their brand name for a specified period of time. They are allowed this exclusivity in order to recoup their expenses in bringing the drug to market. This is called the patent period. After the patent period runs out, however, the door is open for other drug manufacturers to produce and sell the same active ingredient in a medication, but under the generic name, rather than the brand name. And once a medication is available generically, the price usually goes down, sometimes quite significantly.

An obvious question that most people ask is, **"Do generics work just as well as the brand-name product?"**

The answer is "yes", except in only a few cases, which will be explained in a bit. When allowing generic drug manufacturers to make the generic form of medication, the manufacturer must prove to the FDA that the active ingredient in their drug works the same as (or is bioequivalent to) the branded medication. Although the generic formulation may have different inactive ingredients (in other words, fillers), the strength, dose form (such as tablet, capsule, syrup), and route (for example, oral, rectal, intravenous) must be identical. Because of these requirements, you can be assured that generics *are* just as effective, but usually *much* cheaper (an average of 80% less expensive) than the original brand-name products.

Now, what about those one or two generic medications that we mentioned that aren't necessarily as good as the brand-name products? Some examples of these exceptions to the generic rule are levothyroxine (Synthroid), Digoxin, and warfarin (Coumadin). The technical term to describe these types of medications is that they have a "narrow therapeutic index". In other words, even a small variation in dosage can have a large impact on the body's physical function.

So, when it comes to these types of medications, what should you do? You should either: a) choose the brand-name product, and make sure to have it dispensed on every refill; or b) choose the generic version, but insist on the **same generic manufacturer** on every refill of your prescription. Whichever way you choose, you will be consuming the same amount of the active ingredient from month to month, and, therefore, should expect to see the same results from the medication.

Combination products

Combination products are those such as Tenoretic (atenolol plus chlorthalidone) or Diovan HCT (valsartan plus hydrochlorothiazide). These products and others like them have been developed to increase compliance with taking medications.

Why? Because, believe it or not, some people take upwards of 20 or 30 doses of medication per day! The number of pills that they consume can leave them feeling frustrated and, in some cases, the person may make a conscious decision to not take them, simply because there are too many to swallow. By taking a combination product of two different medications, which would otherwise have to be taken individually, the "pill burden" decreases, which may increase compliance.

With increased compliance (that is, taking your medications as prescribed) comes better health. That said, however, this "convenience factor" comes at a price, and the price can be quite substantial. For the folks who are more concerned about the cost of their medications than they are about the quantity of medications, taking the generic formulation of *each* component of the combination medication may be a better alternative. The difference in cost can really add up!

Don't take unnecessary medication

It's unfortunate, but true, that some people use medications that are unnecessary or that can even cause them harm. These medications may be over-the-counter products, herbal remedies, supplements, or even prescription medications. Okay, I know you may be thinking, **"How can I be on an unnecessary medication if my doctor or doctors have prescribed them for me?"** I can only state, based on my experience as a Clinical Pharmacist, is that this does happen, unfortunately, and that it happens too often.

Let's say, for instance, that you have medications prescribed by more than one practitioner, and that, for some reason, these professionals or their practice offices aren't communicating with each other about what they are prescribing. Or, you might simply forget to inform a physician about all current medications during your office visit. When these situations occur, you have a greater chance of being prescribed unnecessary medications. For example, you may be prescribed a medication that interacts with another medication you are already taking, or even treating the same medical condition twice, once by each doctor.

Although these can be scary scenarios, you need not fear! This is where your pharmacist comes into the picture. We as Clinical Pharmacists, especially regarding the management of medications for seniors, use our medication expertise to review your medication list and health conditions to ensure that all your medications are needed, safe for you, carry the least amount of side effects, and are working appropriately to improve your health condition. In almost every case, we can save you money by decreasing the number of medications or over-the-counter formulations that you are taking, which, in the long run, can keep you out of the hospital, enhance your health, and, ultimately, save you money by avoiding inpatient admissions.

Split tablets correctly

Another possible way to save money is to work with your physician or pharmacist in regards to splitting tablets correctly. For instance, perhaps your dose of Drug A is 40mg, but your physician writes you a prescription for 80mg tablets, and tells you to take ½ tablet daily. Sometimes this approach can save you money! All you need to do is talk with your pharmacist, to find out if this will work with your specific medication, and, if so, you can then ask your doctor to write you a prescription for the more affordable tablet.

Manufacturer coupons

Some manufacturers of branded products will offer coupons on their websites, in order to encourage patients to buy their branded products rather than the cheaper generic alternatives. To see if coupons are available, simply go onto the Internet, search the web for the drug manufacturer, then enter the search term "coupons" on their website, and see what pops up.

Drug companies' patient assistance programs

Some drug companies have programs through which they will provide medications for free or at a discounted rate to patients who qualify (usually that means they are eligible based on income). You just need to do a little research to find out if you qualify, and if the manufacturer of your medication offers this type of program. If research feels like more than you can handle on your own, ask your health care provider if a medical social worker, a patient liaison, or an elder ombudsperson is available to assist.

As you can now see, there are safe ways that you can save some of your hard earned cash. You simply have to know about the options, as we've presented them here, and continue to do your research.

OVER-THE-COUNTER (OTC) AND HERBAL SUPPLEMENTS

Unless you are restricted to using mail-order purchases to obtain your prescriptions, and/or you **never** purchase over-the-counter medications, I would venture to say that you have had the complicated experience of standing in the middle of the over-the-counter (OTC) section of your local Pharmacy and trying to choose a product. It makes even my head spin, and I'm a Pharmacist!

I always wonder what the lay public must be thinking when having to decide which product they should pick up and take to the checkout counter. Are they confused? Are they wondering which product is better than another? Perhaps they are concerned about whether the medication will interact with their prescription medications, or, worse yet, they might not even be thinking along these lines.

Whatever their thoughts, I only know that I see a lot of "blank stares" from customers as I look down these aisles; therefore, the focus of this chapter is to give the reader a little bit of knowledge on the most common items purchased in the over-the-counter and herbal supplement aisles.

In this day and age, the information that is readily available online leads many to "self-treat" with over-the-counter and herbal supplements without discussing it with their doctors, practitioners, or pharmacists. Many people are under the impression that, because something can be purchased at a store or pharmacy without a prescription, or because it's labeled "natural", it's safe. In reality, there are many opportunities for drug interactions and side effects with over-the-counter and herbal supplements, so let's get started!

We are only skimming the surface here on *the most common issues to consider*. This should in no way be considered the final authority on OTC and supplement safety, as it depends on your physical and medical history. **It is always a good idea to check with your physician or local pharmacist on safe OTC and supplement choices.**

First, let's go through some questions and answers regarding the basic information that consumers should know:

In the U.S., how do medications get approval to be sold over-the-counter (OTC)?

In general, OTC medications start out as prescription medication and are only changed to OTC status if there is an application submitted by the manufacturer to the Food and Drug Association (FDA. Once this occurs, the FDA will evaluate all of the available data on the medication to see:
- If the active ingredient is SAFE
- If the active ingredient is EFFECTIVE (in other words, asking, "does it work?")
- If the labeling can be written in such a way that the general consumer can safely self-prescribe and self-administer the product, without the input of a medical professional

Are "natural" products (vitamins, minerals, herbal supplements) safer than pharmaceuticals?

Anything that you put into your body, whether medication, herbs, food, or drink, has the opportunity to cause a reaction, good, bad, or neutral. For instance, think about cabbage. Not everyone feels this way, but some people love cooked cabbage! However, cabbage lovers around the world know that if you eat too much, or, for some, even the smallest amount, you most likely will experience burping and/or flatulence. This is simply a chemical reaction: the ingestion of a product resulting in a fairly harmless physical consequence. "natural" products are no different.

To answer the earlier question about whether natural products are safe, the answer is "maybe". It all depends on your individual body's reaction, your current physical health, and the other medications that you may be taking.

In summary, remember that OTC products, including vitamins, minerals, and supplements **should** be considered medications. As mentioned at the beginning of this section, whenever you put something, even food, into your body, there is always a chemical reaction of some sort. It is no different with vitamins, minerals, and supplements. They have the ability to interact with other medications you may be taking, can interfere with certain disease states that you may have, and can potentially be toxic to your system.

How do you safeguard yourself against negative outcomes? Two simple steps: First, make sure to tell your doctor about each and every medication, OTC product, vitamin, mineral, and supplement you are taking. Second, find a Clinical Pharmacist to review all of these products and your individual health conditions, as they are the most knowledgeable health professional when it comes to seniors and their medications.

CONVERSATIONS WITH YOUR HEALTHCARE PROVIDER(S)

When you're a patient with a chronic condition, there are certain things you can do to get the best care from your providers. The number one point to remember is that **you are the captain of your healthcare team.** Your doctors, nurses, and therapists all work for you. Of course, you need to cooperate with the treatments they prescribe; however, they can do their best for you when you step up and become an active player. Coping with a chronic disease or disability can be overwhelming at times. It's often easy to overlook some of the simplest and smartest things you can do to help yourself.

Ask questions.

Plan your questions in advance. When you think of one, write it down. In fact, start a diary to keep a record of your symptoms, side effects, all the medications you take, and most important, your questions. Plan to ask questions about what to expect.

Don't be afraid to ask, "Why?"

Bring your medication journal to your appointments so that you don't forget anything. Then, write down the answers your health care providers give you. If you don't have time to write it all down during the appointment, make notes immediately afterward while the information is still fresh in your mind. There's a lot to keep track of, so keep a written record of everything, or ask someone to go to visits with you. To download templates or purchase a **MedTracker** journal visit www.pillboxtalk.com

If you don't understand the answers, speak up!

It's true that healthcare professionals are busy and often in a hurry, but it's part of their job to listen to you and give you the information you need. Keep in mind that you need to understand your treatment plan so that you can do your part. So ask questions, and keep on asking until you understand.

In an examination room, it's tempting to say what you think the healthcare professional wants to hear, or to say that you're doing better than you really are. However, this is the time to provide complete information about everything that you are feeling and thinking regarding your health! Talk about what is changing, what is better, and what is worse.

Tell your healthcare provider about other conditions you may have, and about all the medicines you are taking.

If you think a prescription medication may be causing a problem, or if you're having trouble affording your medication, mention it. There may be a different medication you can try.

Also, be honest about your health habits. If you miss taking your medication, say so. Be truthful on exactly how much and how often you smoke, drink, and exercise, and what and when you eat. Say something if you have been feeling depressed or anxious.

A healthcare professional can only give you the best treatment—the treatment developed especially for you—if he or she has complete and correct information.

Tell each and every health care provider you see about the other healthcare professionals you are also seeing.

Whether you're receiving acupuncture, physical therapy, chiropractic care, therapeutic massage, or other treatments, each player on the team needs to know the big picture to provide the best care for you. Let them all know if you are taking herbal supplements or vitamins, or if you are on a special diet, whether for health reasons or by personal choice. You are the only person who knows everything that is going on with you, so it's your job to keep everyone on the team informed.

To summarize, the healthcare team consists of providers such as physicians, nurses, pharmacists and case managers, support staff, and most importantly, you, the patient. By working together, this team can play a significant role in improving appropriate medication use. And so the involvement of the entire team is vital to reduce the risk of medication-related problems.

Conversations with Your Physician

Your primary care provider (PCP) is your generalist, the person who you should see regularly. Often, the PCP can then refer you to specialists, depending on your health care needs. For example, someone with a diagnosis of diabetes could easily be followed by their PCP if they are otherwise healthy. In many cases, however, diabetic patients are referred to endocrinologists to manage their diabetes if complex factors and circumstances are present. Another example would be referral to a cardiologist if you have recently had a heart attack or stroke.

It's important, anytime you see a specialist outside of your PCP appointments, that you ensure that all of the information collected and shared with you during that appointment is also sent to your PCP for a complete care model. If there is simply too much information to convey in the appointment, consider asking each provider about a signed medical release of information form, which he or she can use to request records from another provider(s).

Conversations with Your Pharmacist

Each time you get a prescription filled in the United States, whether in a retail store or through a mail-order pharmacy, a licensed pharmacist is there to check that it is the right medication for you and your health conditions. The Community or Retail Pharmacist is available to you within a traditional, physical pharmacy setting. Their main objectives are to ensure that you are given the correct medication for a specific purpose, and to ensure there are no known interactions with your other medications or health conditions. They are accessible to you for a face-to-face consultation, and are often more readily available than your own physician, which makes them among the most trusted professionals available.

The Mail Order Pharmacist conducts the same process as the Community Pharmacist; however, you never see them! That's because they work in what is referred to as a "closed-door pharmacy", which only fills prescriptions delivered to you by mail. Mail order pharmacy has gained popularity over the years with employer groups, because it saves money on medications necessary for their employees' chronic conditions. Yet many patients don't realize that this pharmacist is also readily available to answer questions over the phone.

Your Clinical Pharmacist is also a licensed pharmacist, who has additional certification and training as a medication expert and years of advanced training about how medications can work to improve senior health, specifically. In addition, your Clinical Pharmacist is specially trained to help you use your medications correctly in the home setting. As a home-care model begins to expand, the Clinical Pharmacist will take the time to ensure all medications (prescription, over-the-counter, or herbal) are reviewed, regardless of where they were filled (mail order versus retail pharmacy) or who wrote the prescription (PCP versus specialist).

Conversations with Your Support System

It's important to involve your family members and friends in your healthcare decisions for several reasons. First, it's always nice to have extra moral support when you are first diagnosed with a chronic condition. Having support will enable you to make the best decisions when it comes to how you will modify your life, based on the medications or on the dietary or other changes you will need to make to your current lifestyle. Second, it's important that your friends and family members know what to do on your behalf, in case you are unable to make decisions for yourself.

Many people assume that they would only be unable to make decisions if they were badly hurt in an accident or fall; however, older adults may start developing memory problems fairly early on, and it can become confusing to everyone involved if medical decisions are not made in advance, in writing. For most people, it will be a relief to know that the decisions made tomorrow were carefully thought out, according to their wishes, and with the best of intentions. (Note: Discussion of end-of-life care and directives, of a healthcare proxy, and of power of attorney are beyond the scope of this book; however, many resources and workshops are available through other sources, such as local agencies, community centers or churches. Books on these topics are also widely available.)

Today, there are many options for elders who choose to stay at home, also known as "aging in place". Ensuring that you have the best in-home care providers if you need assistance is essential. Most elders will also rely on family members and friends at some point to provide needed assistance. However, if the care you receive starts to become a daily necessity, getting help from outside your established social support circle is usually necessary.

When seeking professional support, there are two main types of In-Home Care Providers, namely, either Medical or Non-Medical Healthcare providers. Depending on the state where you reside, there are different definitions of each; however, in general, the following applies:

- **Non-Medical Home Health Providers** are only allowed to assist you basic with activities of daily living, such as showering, meal preparation and running errands. They are not allowed to fill your pill boxes or to manage your medications for you.
- **Medical Home Health Providers** are licensed health care providers (such as Nurses, Social Workers,

Occupational Therapists, Pharmacists), who can usually do everything the Non-Medical Home Health Provider does, in addition to managing your medications and making assessments of your limitations and activities of daily living.

The most recognized professional in this setting is the Certified Geriatric Care Manager. These professionals have specialized training and certification in caring for individuals who have been diagnosed with advanced diseases such as Alzheimer's or Parkinson's disease, while those patients continue to live in their own homes. They are truly the experts in home-based care, and they are a great asset to your healthcare team.

It can be hard to keep track of all the advice you receive, and sometimes you'll need to do some follow up on your own. Again, bringing a family member or friend along on your appointments or to the hospital can make you feel more comfortable and more confident, and can help you to have a better conversation with your healthcare provider. Your family member or friend—a person who knows what your day-to-day life is like—can help you to follow through with your treatment and to manage your care once you leave the office or the hospital.

Keep in mind that your health care team is there to help you. This means that you need to let everyone on the team know what is working for you and what is not. Talk to each one of them openly. If you are not comfortable with someone and feel that you can't talk to him or her about your health care needs, or you are not getting the care and attention you need, you could be better off making a change of provider, no matter how difficult it may seem. Again, family and friends, or another trusted provider can provide useful perspectives.

To summarize, if you have a chronic disease or disability that requires you to see health care providers often, you must take the responsibility to follow the treatments you and your providers have worked out together. So step up. Ask questions. Educate yourself. Tell your health care team everything, and keep everyone on your team connected. Network with others. You'll get better care and feel better about it, too!

ASK THE PHARMACIST: EXPERTISE FROM A BOARD CERTIFIED GERIATRIC PHARMACIST

How do I know I'm properly taking my medications as prescribed by my doctor?

It's always important to check with your pharmacist or healthcare provider when a new medication is prescribed, in order to ensure that you understand how to take it properly and that there are no extra precautions given your current medication regimen. Here are some general tips when taking your medications, whether by mouth or other means of administration:

1. Taking medications by mouth
    - It's best to take medications by mouth with a full glass of water.
    - Some medications should be taken with food to avoid stomach upset; however, some are absorbed better with an empty stomach.
    - Always check the label, and when in doubt, contact your pharmacist.

2. Using eye drops
    - Wash your hands
    - Tilt your head back, and, with your index finger, pull the lower eyelid away from the eye to form a pouch.
    - Drop the medication into the pouch and gently close the eye for at least 30 seconds.
    - Avoid touching the applicator tip to any surface (including the eye), and wash your hands after applying the medication.

3. Using eye ointments
    - Wash your hands, then tilt your head back and, with your index finger, pull the lower eyelid away from the eye to form a pouch.
    - Squeeze a thin strip of ointment into the pouch and gently close the eye for at least 30 seconds.
    - Avoid touching the applicator tip to any surface (including the eye) and wash your hands after applying the medication.

4. Using nasal sprays
    - Blow your nose gently, with head upright, then spray medication into each nostril as directed.
    - Inhale briskly while squeezing the bottle quickly and firmly.
    - To clean the applicator after administration; you can rinse the tip with hot water (make sure no water goes inside the bottle) and dry with a clean tissue or cloth.
    - Remember to replace the cap after use.

5. Using ear drops
    - Wash your hands, then lie down, or tilt your head so that your ear faces up.
    - Gently pull the earlobe up and back to straighten the ear canal, and drop the medicine into the ear canal. (Note: For children, you pull down and back.)
    - You can use a sterile cotton plug to prevent the medicine from running out. Avoid touching the applicator tip to any surface including the ear

6. Using suppositories
    - Wash your hands, remove foil wrapper from the individual suppository and moisten it with water or petroleum jelly.
    - Lie down on your side, and push the suppository well into the rectum with your index finger.
    - If the suppository is too soft to insert because the storage temperature was too warm, then before removing it from the foil applicator, chill a wrapped suppository in the refrigerator for 30 minutes, or hold a wrapped suppository under cold running water.

7. Using vaginal applicators
    - Wash your hands, then put the appropriate medication into the applicator provided. Lie down on your back with your knees drawn up to the chest.
    - Insert the applicator into the vagina as far as it can go without using force. Release the medicine by pushing the plunger on the applicator, and then remove the applicator.
    - Clean the applicator with soap and warm water and wash your hands again.

What are some common side effects seen with medications, and what should I look for?

When you receive counseling on a new medication, the pharmacist should always inform you about the medication's common side effects, and about what to do if you experience these yourself. While most side effects may go away as your body adjusts to the medication, if they continue to bother you, always check with your healthcare provider or pharmacist. In general, here are some common side effects that we are asked about as pharmacists, as well as some general suggestions to consider.

1. Allergic reaction
   - If you develop a rash after taking a new medication (as evidenced by a rash, shortness of breath, dizziness, confusion, or any other distressing symptoms), you should immediately stop taking it and call your physician for further advice.
   - If you develop shortness of breath after taking a new medication, you should immediately stop taking it. Go to the nearest emergency room, taking the medication with you, or call 911.

2. Rash
   - Minor skin rashes can often be treated by applying over-the-counter hydrocortisone cream or taking diphenhydramine (Benadryl) by mouth. Note that this medication itself can cause significant drowsiness, so follow the directions and precautions on the label.

- Using a moisturizing lotion after bathing or washing hands can prevent dry skin.
- Protect the rash from sun exposure as well, and avoid extra hot showers.
- Significant rashes, such as those experienced due to an allergy to sulfa drugs, require a physician to evaluate for recommendation.

3. Nausea and/or vomiting
    - If you are undergoing chemotherapy, talk to your physician or pharmacist about available medications to prevent or reduce associated nausea or vomiting.
    - If appropriate, take medications with food to avoid stomach irritation.
    - Eat smaller, more frequent meals throughout the day.

4. Upset stomach
    - Sip small amounts of soda or sparkling water, and eat dry toast or crackers.
    - Avoid taking antacids unless recommended by your physician.
    - If appropriate, take medications with food to avoid stomach upset.

5. Constipation
    - Drink plenty of water and ensure your diet consists of high-fiber (such as vegetables or bran) and avoid fatty foods.
    - Exercise daily, as appropriate to your level of fitness and your doctor's advice.

- For serious constipation, consider adding a stool softener or gentle laxative to your medication regimen, as approved by your physician.

6. Diarrhea
    - Diarrhea caused by a new medication (such as an antibiotic), and usually occurs within the first week of starting the medication.
    - It should resolve on its own; however, taking an over-the-counter probiotic can also help alleviate the issue, if it is related to antibiotic use.
    - If the diarrhea lasts more than a few days, or if it becomes a significant problem, then it's important to call or to visit your physician, particularly to prevent dehydration.

7. Dizziness or lightheadedness
    - Sit up slowly when lying down, and stand up slowly from a seated position.
    - If you feel dizzy or lightheaded after taking a medication, it's important not to drive or operate any mechanical devices.
    - If the dizziness persists, it's important to contact your physician to evaluate your medications and the current dose.

8. Drowsiness
    - Avoid drinking any alcoholic beverages when using a medication that is known to cause drowsiness (for example, diphenhydramine Benadryl™).

- If a new medication is causing you to feel sleepy, it's important not drive or operate any mechanical devices.

9. Dry mouth
    - Rinse your mouth throughout the day with warm salt water.
    - Suck on sugarless hard candies, lozenges, or crushed ice to cool your mouth and give it moisture.
    - Chew sugarless gum to stimulate saliva, or try slippery elm or licorice tea to lubricate the mouth.
    - Sip water throughout the day, and wear lip balm.
    - If none of these remedies work for you, ask your physician to prescribe a product or mouth rinse for you to treat your chronic dry mouth.

10. Dry skin
    - Use gentle soaps and detergents (dye- and fragrance-free).
    - Use hand and body lotion after taking a bath or washing hands.

11. Gas or bloating
    - Use an over-the-counter product such as simethicone.
    - Use an over-the-counter probiotic supplement, or eat plain yogurt.

12. Chest pain or tightness
    - If you experience tightness in the chest or throat after taking a new medication, you should

immediately stop taking it and call your physician for further advice.
- If the chest pain is significant or does not go away, immediately go to the nearest emergency room or call 911.

13. Headache
    - Rest in a quiet, dark room, with your eyes closed and cold washcloth over the eyes or forehead.
    - Massage the base of the skull with your thumbs, and also massage both temples gently.
    - Check with your pharmacist to see which over-the-counter remedies are appropriate for you.
    - To prevent headaches from getting worse, avoid trigger foods such as caffeine, chocolate, red wine, citrus fruit, food additives, cheese, and vinegar.

14. Low blood sugar (hypoglycemia)
    - Avoid letting your blood sugar go lower than 70 mg/dl.
    - Call your physician if any of your blood sugar indicators or tests are too low, or if you notice any of these symptoms: irritability, nervousness, pale skin, trembling or rapid heartbeat, blurred vision, fatigue, confusion, slowed reaction time, or loss of consciousness.
    - If you are a diabetic, it's important to keep items with you, such as hard candies, glucose tablets, or fruit juice, to avoid letting your blood sugar go too low.

15. Low blood pressure (hypotension)
    - Take your medication when sitting down.
    - When first starting a new medication, be careful when standing up from a seated position.

16. Unable to sleep (insomnia)
    - Keep the bedroom dark.
    - Only use the bedroom to sleep, not for any other activity.
    - Remove any light sources or noises that may interfere with your sleep pattern.
    - Avoid caffeine or sugary foods or drinks before bedtime or late in the day.
    - Exercise or get plenty of activity during the daytime.
    - Discuss your current medication regimen with your pharmacist, and move any medications administration to morning rather than evening, if possible.

17. Nasal congestion or dryness
    - Saline nose drops and/or a light coating of petroleum jelly on the nostrils can alleviate most nasal dryness issues.

18. Sun sensitivity
    - Some medications can make your skin more sensitive to the sun, so it's important to check the label and to ask your pharmacist whenever starting a new medication.

- Wear sunscreen, and avoid long exposure to the sun.
- Wear sunglasses and protective clothing.

19. Weight gain
    - Some medications can cause weight gain, so it's important to ask your pharmacist and read the label whenever starting a new medication.
    - Exercise and improve eating habits, such as incorporating more vegetables and fiber into diet, and avoiding fatty foods.

Take Part in Decisions about Your Treatment

Don't be afraid to "bother" your doctor with your concerns and questions. You may want to write down questions to ask at your next visit to the doctor. By taking time to ask questions now, you may avoid problems later. Bring a friend or family member with you when you visit your doctor. They can help you remember what the doctor said and what questions you need to ask. Having someone along that you trust can help you make better choices, especially if you are not feeling well and/or distracted. You can also talk to your pharmacist about the medications you are taking.

Know Your Medications
- Keep an up-to-date list.
- Take a current medication list to all doctors appointments.
- Talk with your doctor **and** your pharmacist about all medications.
- Take medications as directed **and** check expiration dates.
- Store medications properly.

Tips for Safe Medication Adherence
(Or, Dos and Don'ts for Medication Safety)

DO read the label carefully, including the prescription label or any label that comes on the vitamin/nutritional supplement, herbal product, or non-prescription medication.
DO tell your doctor and pharmacist about any drug or food allergies that you may have.
DO take your medication exactly as your doctor prescribes.
DO make sure that each of your doctors has a complete list of all your medications including prescription, over-the-counter, vitamin or nutritional supplements, and herbals products.
DO consider using one pharmacy for all your medications, so that the pharmacist can help you to keep track of your medications and screen your medications for drug interactions.
DO ask your doctor or pharmacist to help you make a schedule to use to take your medications daily, so that you will know what medications to take at what time of day, and whether you should take medications together.
DO make sure that everyone you live with knows what medications you take and when you are supposed to take them.
DO keep track of any side effects that you may be having, and notify your doctor about these immediately.
DO go through your medicine cabinet at least once a year, and get rid of old or expired medications.
DO have all your medications reviewed by your doctor at least once a year.

DON'T take someone else's medications.

DON'T combine prescription and over-the-counter medications or herbal, vitamin, or nutritional supplements without first checking with your doctor or pharmacist.

DON'T stop taking a medication or change how much you take or how often you take it without first checking with your doctor.

DON'T use medications beyond their expiration dates.

DON'T crush, break, or chew tablets or capsules unless your doctor or pharmacist says it is okay. Some medications don't work unless they are swallowed whole. If you cannot swallow a medication, ask your pharmacist or doctor if there are other dosage forms that you could use.

Last, But Not Least: *Always* Ask Your Doctor or Pharmacist About New Medications

1. **What am I taking?**
2. **What is it for?**
3. **When do I take it?**
4. **Are there any side effects?**
5. **Are there any special instructions?**

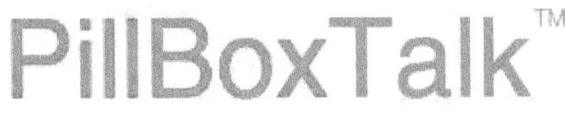

PillBoxTalk™

answers to your medication questions

www.pillboxtalk.com

Meet the Pharmacist

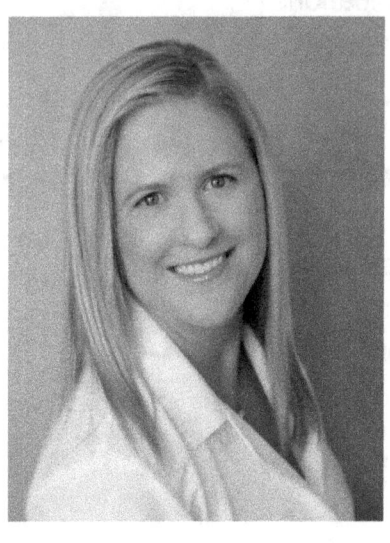

"A successful partnership between the healthcare provider and patient is one in which each is aware of their role in preventing and managing medication-related problems."

Dr. Stephanie Matinpour, PharmD, BCGP

Dr. Stephanie Matinpour is a Board-Certified Geriatric Pharmacist, who received her Doctor of Pharmacy degree from the University of the Pacific School of Pharmacy and completed her general Pharmacy Practice Residency in San Diego, CA.

Dr. Matinpour is a Senior Care Pharmacy expert and founder of the PillBoxTalk Foundation, providing medication safety and educational workshops to Geriatric Care Managers and caregivers. Her focus is on working with those who manage patients with chronic conditions and multiple medication issues. She takes the mystery and myth out of medication-related questions by practicing evidence-based medicine, and provides the tools you need to be your own, best patient advocate. Working in the pharmacy field for the past 20 years, Dr. Matinpour has studied various areas of pharmacy and has worked in multiple medical disciplines.

Dr. Matinpour was a 2012 ASCP Foundation Entrepreneurship Grant recipient. She has worked in various pharmacy settings including Hospital Pharmacy, Community Pharmacy, and, primarily, as a Clinical Pharmacist, providing medication therapy management for those patients on multiple medications. Dr. Matinpour also has extensive experience with medication safety guidelines and regulatory requirements for assuring appropriate pharmaceutical care.

Dr Matinpour is a licensed Pharmacist in the State of California and has served as an adjunct professor at the University of the Pacific School of Pharmacy and as a volunteer faculty member at the University of San Diego Skaggs School of Pharmacy.

Learn more about avoiding medication related problems and tools to be your best medication advocate at
www.pillboxtalk.com

References

1. Arch Intern Med 2004;164:1567-72
2. REFERENCES: APhA Questions to ask your Pharmacist
3. Gurwitz J., Monane M., Monane S., Avorn J. Long-Term Care Quality Letter. Brown University. 1995; Murphy J. Senate Special Committee on Aging. quoted in The Washington Post, May 30, 1999.
4. Levy, H.B. Self-administered medication-risk questionnaire in an elderly population. Ann Pharmacother 2003; 37:982-7.
5. Elizabeth Oyekan, PharmD, FCSHP, Ananda Nimalasuriya, MD, John Martin, MD, Ron Scott, MD, R James Dudl, MD, and Kelley Green, RN, PhD The B-Smart Appropriate Medication-Use Process Perm J. 2009 Winter; 13(1): 62–69.
6. Cross, A. J., et.al. (2020). Interventions for improving medication-taking ability and adherence in older adults prescribed multiple medications. Cochrane Database of Systematic Reviews, (5). /doi/10.1002/14651858.CD012419.pub2/epdf/full
7. Sabaté, Eduardo, and Eduardo Sabaté, eds.(2003) Adherence to long-term therapies: evidence for action. World Health Organization..
8. National Council on Disability. Best Practices for Accessible Prescription Drug Labeling.
9. Lindauer, Allison, Kathryn Sexson, and Theresa A. Harvath. "Medication management for people with dementia." AJN The American Journal of Nursing 117.2 (2017): 60-64.
10. Meducation, Adult. "Improving medication adherence in older adults." American Society on Aging and American Society of Consultant Pharmacists Foundation (2006).
11. Institute on Aging. A Caregiver's role in safe medication management for seniors
12. Health insurance counseling and advocacy program. (2018) Medicare Counseling
13. U.S. National Library of Medicine: MedlinePlus. Storing your medicines.
14. California Drug Take-Back Program. https://www.takebackdrugs.org
15. U.S. Food & Drug Administration: Where and How to Dispose of Unused Medicines. Accessed 20 May 2020.

16. U.S. Food & Drug Administration: Drug Disposal: Drug Take Back Locations. Accessed 20 May 2020.
17. U.S. Food & Drug Administration: Disposal of Unused Medicines: What You Should Know. Accessed 20 May 2020.
18. U.S. Food & Drug Administration. Safely Using Sharps (Needles and Syringes) at Home, at Work and on Travel.
19. https://www.usp.org/health-quality-safety/usp-pictograms
20. *Vial of Life Website. www.vialoflife.com*
21. http://www.nationalhealthcouncil.org/NHC_Files/files/healthcareteam.pdf
22. https://www.calrecycle.ca.gov/HomeHazWaste/medications/household
23. https://www.calrecycle.ca.gov/HomeHazWaste/Sharps/
24. https://www.fda.gov/drugs/safe-disposal-medicines/disposal-unused-medicines-what-you-should-know
25. https://www.fda.gov/drugs/drug-information-consumers/buying-using-medicine-safely
26. https://www.fda.gov/drugs/drug-information-consumers/tips-seniors
27. https://www.aginglifecare.org/ALCA/About_Aging_Life_Care/Consumer_Resources/ALCA/About_Aging_Life_Care/Consumer_Resources.aspx?hkey=a7e6c04d-6e44-4d96-adcb-2fb673870494

www.ingramcontent.com/pod-product-compliance
Lightning Source LLC
Chambersburg PA
CBHW060435220526
45465CB00008B/3147